HOW TO SUPPRESS APPETITE

How to Suppress Appetite and Helps You Lose Weight

Arthur L. Johnson

Table of Contents

CHAPTER 1

TEN NATURAL WAYS TO REDUCE APPETITE

A food, supplement, or other method that prevents a person from feeling hungry is known as an appetite suppressant. Some methods work better than others to reduce appetite.

Pill manufacturers make exaggerated claims regarding their products' capacity to suppress appetite and encourage weight loss. However, the National Institutes of Health (NIH) reports that these pills frequently come with harmful side effects and that their effectiveness is unknown.

Instead, a person can use a variety of risk-free and healthy natural methods to suppress or lose appetite.

In this article, we give a rundown of proof based techniques that an individual can use to stifle their hunger without the requirement for diet pills. Additionally, we talk about which foods work best to suppress appetite.

Natural appetite suppressants a person can use the ten methods that are supported by evidence to curb their appetite and avoid overeating:

1. Eat more protein and healthy fats Eating foods that are high in protein or fat can stop you from feeling hungry and make you feel fuller for longer.

Hunger is not satisfied equally by all foods. Protein and some fats work better than carbohydrates to satisfy hunger and keep people feeling full for longer.

Proteins and healthy fats can help a person control their appetite by replacing some carbohydrate sources.

Dietary Guidelines for Americans suggests the following high-protein foods:

Lean meats, eggs, beans, and peas, soy products, Greek yogurt, and lean meats. The guidelines also recommend that healthy fats come from natural sources like olive oil, nuts, and seeds.

2. Drink water before every meal. According to Trusted Source, drinking a large glass of water right before a meal makes you feel fuller, more satisfied, and less hungry.

Another study looked at 50 overweight women's appetite and found that drinking 1.5 liters of water a day for eight weeks reduced appetite and weight, as well as increased fat loss.

A soup starter might also make you feel fuller. According to a 2007 study, people who ate with a liquid starter reported feeling fuller right away.

3. Eat more foods with a lot of fiber because fiber doesn't break down as quickly as other foods do, so it stays in your body longer. People feel fuller for the rest of the day as a result of this, which also slows digestion.

According to research, fiber may be able to suppress appetite.

Diets high in fiber are also linked to lower rates of obesity.

Then again, another review found that bringing additional fiber into the eating regimen was powerful in under portion of the examinations they checked out.

To determine which sources of fiber are most effective at suppressing appetite, additional research is required.

Foods with a lot of fiber are good for you:

Vegetables, whole grains, beans, pulses, apples, avocados, almonds, and chia seeds Exercise before eating is another healthy and effective way to suppress your appetite.

According to a 20-study review, exercise, particularly high-intensity workouts, immediately suppresses appetite hormones.

They discovered higher levels of "fullness hormones" like PPY and GLP-1 and lower levels of ghrelin, a hormone that makes us hungry.

5. Drink Yerba Maté tea

Research shows that high-intensity exercise and a tea made from the Ilex paraguariensis plant called Yerba Maté can help reduce appetite and improve mood. Online purchasing is available for Yerba Maté.

6. Switch to dark chocolate. Compared to milk chocolate, dark chocolate has been shown to reduce appetite. According to a Trusted Source study, snacking on dark chocolate instead of milk chocolate reduced subsequent calorie intake.

7. Eat some ginger. According to Trusted Source, consuming a small amount of ginger powder has been shown to

reduce appetite and increase fullness. This may be because ginger powder stimulates the digestive system. Since this was a small study, additional research is required to verify this effect. Online retailers offer ginger powder for purchase.

8. Eat a lot of calorie-dense foods when dieters cut back on their overall food intake, it can make them hungry. A relapse into binge eating may result from this.

However, dieting does not necessarily necessitate starvation. There are some foods that are low in calories but high in nutrients and energy. These incorporate vegetables, natural products, beans, and entire grains.

A person will still be able to burn more calories than they consume if they consume a large quantity of these foods, which will also prevent the stomach from growing ling.

9. Stress less Comfort eating is different from physical hunger because it is caused by stress, rage, or sadness.

Stress has been linked to an increased desire to eat, binge

eating, and eating innutritious food, according to Research.

According to one review, mindfulness practices and mindful eating may lessen comfort eating and binge eating caused by stress. Stress can also be reduced through regular sleep, social interaction, and time spent relaxing.

10. Mindful eating the brain plays a significant role in determining when and what a person consumes. It's possible that a person will consume less food if they focus on what they're eating rather than watching television while they eat.

People ate 36% more after eating a large meal in the dark, according to research published in the journal Appetite. During meals, paying attention to what you're eating can help you avoid overeating.

According to a different article that was reviewed by, mindfulness may have the potential to lessen the effects of comfort eating and binge eating—two important factors that contribute to obesity.

To reduce appetite, the of the National Institutes of Health recommends using mind-body practices like yoga and meditation.

13 Science-Based Ways to Reduce Hunger and Appetite Everyone is familiar with hunger and appetite.

Even when we aren't aware of it, we navigate these biological processes on a daily basis for the most part.

In general, your body sends signals of hunger and appetite when it needs energy or craves a particular kind of food.

Even though feeling hungry is a normal sign that it's time to eat again, it's not fun to feel hungry all the time, especially after a meal. That could be a sign that you're not eating enough food or that you're not combining foods properly.

You may be wondering how to reduce feelings of hunger throughout the day if you are trying to lose weight, living with certain health conditions, or starting a new meal routine like intermittent fasting.

However, hunger and appetite are complex processes that are influenced by numerous internal and external factors, which can make it challenging to reduce either.

CHAPTER 2

WE'VE COMPILED THIS LIST OF 13 SCIENCE-BACKED WAYS TO HELP YOU FEEL FULLER FOR LONGER.

1. FreshSplash and Getty Images Eat enough protein Protein can make you feel fuller, lower your levels of the hormones that cause hunger, and possibly help you eat less at your next meal.

In a small study with 20 healthy adults who were overweight or obese, people who ate eggs (a food high in protein) for breakfast instead of cereal (a food low in protein) felt more full and had lower levels of hunger hormones.

Drinking a beverage high in protein and fiber 30 minutes before eating pizza appeared to reduce feelings of hunger and the amount of pizza consumed by overweight adults in another study.

Protein's ability to suppress appetite isn't just found in animal products like meat and eggs. Beans and peas, two examples of vegetable proteins, may also be beneficial for reducing food intake and keeping you satisfied.

It is sufficient to provide health benefits to consume protein at a rate of 0.45-0.55 grams per pound (1.0–1.2 grams per kilogram) of body weight, or at least 20%–30% of your total calorie intake. However, there are some studies that suggest as much as 0.55–0.73 grams per pound (1.2–1.6 grams per kilogram) of body weight

However, when it comes to high-protein diets, other studies have found contradictory results.

As a result, it is essential to keep in mind that there may be a different kind of diet that is more in line with your eating habits and preferences.

Summary Protein is a nutrient that makes you feel fuller for longer. There are many reasons why eating enough protein is important, but one of the ways it may help you lose weight is by making you feel fuller.

2. Choose foods high in fiber. Eating a lot of fiber slows down digestion and influences the release of hormones that make you feel fuller and control your appetite.

In addition, fiber aids in the production of short-chain fatty acids in the gut, which are thought to increase feelings of fullness.

When mixed with liquids, viscous fibers like pectin, guar gum, and psyllium thicken and may be particularly filling. Viscous fibers can be found naturally in plant foods, but they are also frequently taken as supplements.

According to a recent study, viscous, fiber-rich legumes like lentils, peas, chickpeas, and beans can even increase feelings of fullness by 31% when compared to similar meals that do not include beans. Whole grains high in fiber can also reduce hunger.

However, some researchers believe it is premature to draw generalizations regarding the connection between dietary fiber and appetite because the methods used in studies examining this relationship have not always been consistent.

However, diets high in fiber have not been linked to many negative effects. Many other beneficial nutrients, such as vitamins, minerals, antioxidants, and beneficial plant compounds, can be found in foods high in fiber.

As a result, following a diet high in fruits, vegetables, beans, nuts, and seeds can also improve health over time. Additionally, the combination of protein and fiber may double the benefits for reducing hunger.

Summary Eating a diet high in fiber can help you eat fewer calories and feel less hungry. It additionally advances long haul wellbeing.

3. Drink a lot of water. Some people have reported feeling less hungry and losing weight after drinking water. Additionally, animal studies have demonstrated that hunger and thirst are frequently misunderstood.

According to a small human study, those who consumed two glasses of water immediately prior to a meal consumed 22% less than those who did not (22%)

Scientists think that drinking about 17 ounces (500 milliliters) of water can stretch the stomach and tell the brain when you're full. This advice might work best if you drink water right before a meal because water passes quickly through the stomach.

It's interesting to note that starting your meal with a soup made with broth may have the same effect. A previous study found that having a bowl of soup before a meal reduced hunger and the amount of calories consumed from the meal by approximately 100 calories.

However, not everyone may experience this. There are a number of factors at play, including genetics, the kind of soup you eat, and others. According to 36, 37, and 38 Trusted Sources, soups with savory umami flavor profiles may be more filling than others.

Although the neurons that control your appetite for both water and food are closely related, there is still a lot to learn about how they interact and why drinking water may also satisfy your hunger or appetite for solid foods (39, 40, 41, and 42).

According to some studies, the state of your thirst and the amount of water you drink appear to have a greater impact on your preferences for particular foods than hunger or the amount of food you consume.

Even though it's important to stay hydrated, you shouldn't drink water instead of eating. In general, drink water whenever you eat or before you sit down to eat. Keep a glass with you at all times.

Summary: Consuming low-calorie beverages or soup before a meal may help you consume fewer calories without feeling full.

4. Pick solids food varieties to tame yearning

Strong calories and fluid calories might influence your craving and your cerebrum's prize framework in an unexpected way.

According to two recent reviews of the literature, solid foods and those with a higher viscosity—also known as thickness—significantly reduced hunger in comparison to thin and liquid foods.

One small study found that people who ate hard foods like white rice and raw vegetables had fewer calories at lunch and at their next meal than people who ate soft foods like risotto and boiled vegetables.

According to another study, those who consumed foods with more complex textures consumed significantly less food overall during the meal.

Chewing solid foods takes longer, which may give the brain more time to process the feeling of fullness. However, soft foods may be easier to overeat because they can be consumed quickly in large bites.

Another theory for why solid foods help you feel fuller longer is that chewing gives them more time to interact with your taste buds, which can help you feel fuller longer.

Try to include a wide range of flavors and textures in your meal to keep you full and get a wide range of nutrients.

Summary Eating foods with a lot of texture rather than calories that are thin or liquid can help you eat less without feeling hungry.

5. Eat mindfully under normal circumstances, your brain

assists your body in determining when you are full or hungry.

Your brain has a harder time recognizing these signals if you eat too quickly or while distracted.

Practicing mindful eating, which emphasizes focusing on the foods in front of you, is one strategy for resolving this issue.

Mindful eating is a way to tap into your internal hunger and satiety cues, such as your thoughts and physical feelings, rather than letting external cues like advertisements or the time of day dictate when you eat.

People who are prone to emotional, impulsive, and reward-driven eating, all of which have an impact on hunger and appetite, may benefit most from practicing mindfulness while eating.

However, when combined with a healthy diet, regular physical activity, and other behavior-focused therapies, it appears that mindful eating works best for reducing food cravings and increasing awareness of food.

Summary it has been demonstrated that mindful eating increases feelings of fullness and reduces hunger. It might also help cut down on emotional eating and calories.

6. Eat slowly when you have a strong appetite or are feeling hungry, it can be easy to eat more than you planned. According to, one way to lessen your propensity to overeat is to eat at a slower pace.

A study found that people who ate faster consumed more food in larger portions and consumed more calories overall.

According to another study, foods consumed slowly are more filling than foods consumed quickly.

Curiously, some fresher exploration even proposes that you're eating rate can influence your endocrine framework, including blood levels of chemicals that cooperate with your stomach related framework and craving and satiety signs, like insulin and pancreatic polypeptide.

Summary Eating slowly could make you feel fuller at the end of a meal and help you eat fewer calories overall.

7. Find out what kind of dinnerware works best for you might have heard that eating from

a smaller plate or a utensil of a certain size can help you eat less.

It's possible that cutting down on the size of your dinnerware will also help you eat smaller meals without even realizing it. You are more likely to overeat when you have more food on a larger plate.

According to some studies, eating with a smaller spoon or fork may not directly affect your appetite, but it may help you eat less by slowing down your eating rate and causing you to take smaller bites.

However, results from other studies have been inconsistent.

A number of personal factors, such as your culture, upbringing, and learned behaviors, influence how the size of your dinnerware affects your hunger levels, according to researchers.

Although the advantages of eating on a smaller plate may have been exaggerated in the past, this does not rule out the possibility of giving it a shot.

Try different sizes of plates and utensils to see if they affect how hungry you are, how hungry you are, or how much you eat overall.

Summary Eating from smaller plates may help you eat less unconsciously without making you feel hungry, but the results can be very different from person to person.

8. Regular exercise is thought to lower the activation of brain regions associated with food cravings, which can lower the desire to consume high-calorie foods and increase the desire to consume low-calorie foods.

Additionally, it boosts feelings of fullness while

simultaneously decreasing levels of hunger hormones.

According to some studies, aerobic and resistance exercise are both equally effective at influencing hormone levels and meal size after exercise.

By and large, practice seems to affect hunger for the vast majority, however it's critical to take note of that reviews have seen a wide fluctuation in the manner people and their craving answer work out.

To put it another way, there is no assurance that everyone will experience the same outcomes.

However, there are numerous advantages to exercise, so it's a good idea to incorporate enjoyable movement into your day.

Summary Aerobic and resistance training both have the potential to boost hormones that make you feel full, which in turn can help you eat less and feel less hungry. Activities with a higher intensity may have the greatest effects.

9. Sleep enough Good sleep may also help reduce hunger and prevent weight gain.

According to 88 and 89 trusted sources, insufficient sleep has been linked to an increase in subjective feelings of hunger, appetite, and food cravings.

Lack of sleep can likewise cause a height in ghrelin — a yearning chemical that increments food consumption and is an indication that the body is eager, as well as the hunger controlling chemical leptin.

The majority of adults require between 7 and 9 hours of sleep, while children and adolescents require between 8 and 12 hours.

Summary: It is likely that getting at least seven hours of sleep each night will help you feel less hungry throughout the day.

10. Keep your stress levels under control Excessive stress is known to raise cortical levels.

High cortical levels are generally thought to increase food cravings and the drive to eat, and they have even been linked to weight gain, despite the fact that its effects can vary from person to person.

Peptide YY (PYY), a hormone that makes you feel

fuller, may also be reduced by stress.

CHAPTER 3

ON THE OTHER HAND, STRESS AFFECTS DIFFERENT PEOPLE IN DIFFERENT WAYS.

According to one study, acute stress actually reduced appetite.

Whether you've seen that you will generally feel hungrier when you're under pressure or frequently end up pressure eating intense circumstances, think about a portion of these strategies to lighten your pressure:

Reduce your stress levels may help reduce cravings, increase fullness, and even protect against depression and obesity. Eat a healthy diet full of foods that help relieve stress. Exercise regularly. Drink green tea. Try yoga or stretching. Limit your intake of caffeine.

11. Consume some ginger for its antioxidant and anti-inflammatory properties.

According to, ginger actually has a reputation for increasing appetite in cancer patients by easing the stomach and reducing nausea.

However, a new benefit that has been added to the list is that it may help alleviate hunger.

In one animal experiment, ginger, peppermint, horse gram, and whey protein were added to a herbal mixture that rats were fed. Although the results cannot be attributed solely to the ginger, the combination was found to assist in appetite regulation and satiety induction.

However, more human studies are required before

definitive conclusions regarding ginger and hunger can be drawn.

Summary Ginger may assist in reducing feelings of hunger in addition to adding flavor and settling your stomach. However, additional research is required to verify this effect.

12. Settle on filling snacks

Eating involves individual decision. Snacks are a part of the daily meal plan for some people, but not for others.

Snacks may be able to help you control your hunger and

appetite levels throughout the day, according to some research.

Choose snacks that are high in the following nutrients to help you feel full and satisfied:

Protein, fiber, healthy fats, complex carbs, and healthy fats A high-protein yogurt, for instance, reduces hunger more effectively than high-fat crackers or chocolate snacks.

In point of fact, consuming a serving of high-protein yogurt in the afternoon not only helps you feel fuller for longer, but it may also help you consume fewer calories later on in the day.

Summary Eating a snack with a lot of protein or fiber will probably make you feel less hungry and may keep you from eating too much at your next meal.

13. Don't starve yourself. There are a lot of biological pathways involved in the complicated relationship between appetite, hunger, and cravings.

According to, researchers are still attempting to determine whether restricting certain foods is an effective strategy for reducing food cravings.

According to, some individuals are more susceptible to

cravings because they tend to experience cravings more frequently.

The majority of people do not need to completely eliminate their favorite foods from their diet. After all, you should and can eat your favorite foods.

If you have a craving for a particular food, try enjoying it in moderation to see if it helps you feel less hungry again.

Summary: Depriving yourself completely of the foods you crave may be more effective at suppressing hunger and cravings than enjoying them in moderation.

In conclusion, appetite and hunger are normal bodily functions.

Ordinarily, they're basically a sign that your body needs energy and now is the ideal time to eat.

During times when you feel like your appetite and hunger are higher than usual, the suggestions presented here are merely a few easy ways to reduce them.

If you've tried these things and still feel hungry more than usual, you might want to talk to a doctor about getting more help controlling your appetite.

Foods that suppress appetite there are some foods that work better than others to suppress appetite, such as:

Consuming honey instead of sugar may reduce appetite.

Foods high in protein and healthy fats. Avocado, beans, nuts, cheese, and lean meats are among these.

Foods high in fiber. Foods high in fiber help people feel fuller for longer. Whole grains, beans, fruits, and vegetables are excellent examples.

According to a 2017 review, pulses like beans, lentils, and

chickpeas can directly increase feelings of fullness and may also reduce subsequent food intake.

Eggs may help you feel fuller longer and less hungry throughout the day because of their high protein and fat content.

In people who aren't used to eating spicy foods, cayenne pepper may make them eat less.

Honey may make people feel fuller for longer by suppressing the hunger hormone ghrelin. Honey should be considered an alternative to sugar.

Outlook Excessively restricting food intake may result in a relapse of overeating. Instead, eating enough of the right foods can help you feel less hungry and less tempted to eat throughout the day.

By eating more protein, fat, and fiber in their meals, people can reduce their appetite. A person may feel fuller for longer if they consume a lot of vegetables and pulses.

To combat unwelcome food cravings, it may also be beneficial to experiment with various spices, such as ginger and cayenne pepper, and to consume tea.

THE END

www.ingramcontent.com/pod-product-compliance
Lightning Source LLC
LaVergne TN
LVHW020011170826
845677LV00022B/2708

* 9 7 9 8 3 6 9 6 9 3 8 3 4 *